Itty Bitty Book About

LOWER BACK PAIN

The Ultimate Self-Help Guide
For Those Seeking Natural Relief

DR. CHARLIE JOHNSON
PHYSICAL THERAPIST

Itty Bitty Book About Lower Back Pain

© 2016 Dr. Charlie Johnson

Book Author and Illustrations: Dr. Charlie Johnson
Book Editor and Photo Credits: Heather Johnson (the lovely wife)
Book & Cover Design: IF Design Graphic Design & Photography,
Ida Fia Sveningsson Konsult

ISBN-13: 9781535348430

Dedication

To my wife, Heather, who has supported me each step of the way... through the good and the bad, the wild and crazy, the late nights and early mornings - you're my biggest fan, rock, and my one true love. Thank you for inspiring me to never give up, encouraging me to chase my dreams, and most of all... always believing in me. Without you I'd be lost... I love you - forever.

To my family, for teaching me the power of hard work and resilience through the rollercoaster of life.

To my mentors, who selflessly shared their stories and devoted their time and resources to teach me, guide me, open doors, build me up and break me down... without a single request for anything in return. You've changed my life.

To my PT friends and colleagues who never settle for anything less than the best, for always asking "why," and for pushing the profession forward.

To all those I have served (my patients) who challenged me, kept me honest, and inspired me to always be my best.

To all those I will serve (future patients)... for allowing me to live out my passion and continue changing lives.

Special thanks to:
Carla Zielinski (my high school guidance counselor)... without you none of this would have been possible. Thank you for believing in me.

Dr. Roger Nelson - for your guidance and support through PT school, mentorship, hand-me-down books, lawn cutting side jobs, and your devotion to our profession. Oh... and endless Five Guys Burgers and yogurt. You'll never be forgotten.

Chad Madden of Madden Physical Therapy who inspired me to open my own practice. Thank you for being a role model... for planting a seed, for challenging me to see the bigger picture, to answer the question of "so what," and showing me the power of hard work, determination, and massive ACTION! I'll pay it forward...

My USC residency mentors & crew... and Emeka. Your passion is unmatched, your drive is never ending, and your persistent quest for greatness is an inspiration to all around you. No matter how far apart... thank you for all you do. Stay Iconoclastic.

And Finally, to you (the reader) for reaching out and searching for answers, for taking control of your health in the pursuit of getting back to the life YOU deserve. Enjoy this "Itty Bitty Book."

Table of Contents

Introduction

Hello everyone,

My name is Dr. Charlie Johnson...a physical therapist specializing in the treatment of lower back pain and sciatica.

Before we get started, I'm going to take a wild guess... I'm guessing that you are reading this book for one of two (or both) reasons:

Reason #1: You, or someone you know, are looking for answers as to what could be causing your lower back pain OR leg pain, numbness and tingling.

Reason #2: Even if you don't care to know what's causing it (you're just sick and tired of dealing with it)... you are looking to find a solution that will put an end to your pain starting today.

If this is the case and you are curious about what may be causing your pain and how you can get rid of it...then this book may just be a lifesaver.

I say *may* be a lifesaver because there are many things that can cause lower back and leg pain, numbness, or tingling.

If treated incorrectly, your symptoms could actually get worse.

That's why we are taking all precautions to make sure this book is right for you.

You see, during my training... I've learned many tips and tricks to help naturally heal lower back pain and sciatica.

In fact, I've traveled from coast to coast (literally) in search of answers to better help people just like you.

The self tests and strategies I share with you in this book are a combination of knowledge from many years of practice and study – specifically designed to help you find out what could be causing your lower back pain and sciatica and relieve it.

Now, while I cannot guarantee that each and every one of these strategies will be useful, I can promise you that they will increase your chance of getting relief from lower back pain and sciatica, while changing the way you think about everyday activities.

In this itty bitty book, you'll learn:

- The "big picture" anatomy of the spine and lower back to help you understand what could be going on.

- What nerves are and how they work.

- The most common causes of lower back pain and sciatica and what they mean for your recovery.

- Self-Movement Tests to help you determine the cause of your lower back pain and/or sciatica.

- My top 3 exercises for the 3 common causes of lower back pain and sciatica.

- Personal exercises I use with my very own clients to help them get "up close and personal" with their lower back pain and sciatica...to help them do more of what helps and less of what hurts.

- Step-by-step instructions to help you create your own "Trouble Tree," pain and problems journal, as well as a body diagram to help record exactly what you're feeling and where you're feeling it.

- Day-2-Day Strategies to help change how you think about everyday activities.

- The latest and greatest research on pain...including tips and tricks to help you better understand why you feel what you feel.

- The 7 must-ask questions before choosing a physical therapist.

- A bullet-proof next step action plan to naturally heal lower back pain and sciatica.

Using the above strategies, people just like you are experiencing natural healing for lower back pain and sciatica. Here's what some of my clients have to say about their success:

" *I had severe back pain on the left hand side that was constant. I had difficulty getting out of bed in the morning and problems getting up from a chair.*

I was told that I had some disc issues in my lower back & needed physical therapy which brought me to Charlie Johnson.

I had 4-5 visits with Charlie who helped me with exercises that would essentially strengthen my core and prevent me from rolling my back. Body presses, backward leg lifts and balancing on an exercise ball a couple times each day in addition to presses every two hours during the work day has helped tremendously.

I am able to get up in the morning and get up from a chair without pain thanks to Charlie's assessment of my situation and development of exercises to alleviate the pain.

Thank you, Charlie!"

– Steve Twersky

" *I want to thank Charlie Johnson for helping to restore this 76 year old body to again being pain-free.*

I was in agony every morning when I arose and was hobbling around a good part of the day. Sometimes I could barely stand for more than a few minutes. I went to an orthopedic surgeon, had all kinds of test done, was on pain pills and finally ended up meeting Charlie Johnson.

After a few weeks of therapy with exercises there and at home, I did a complete turn around. I am presently pain-free in my back, legs and buttocks.

I am now walking on the treadmill almost five miles/day and feel great.

I would highly recommend Charlie and the clinic for many reasons.

They are professional in every way and it was a pleasant experience all around. I would go there again if the occasion arises.

My thanks to Charlie."

– Marcia Plager

" I am a pediatric PT and expect a high level of knowledge, expertise and confidence from the PT that I go to see. Charlie is a great PT. His methods are evidence based. My radiating pain was under control within two visits. He progressed me through treatment by pushing me while also being very conscious of what could flare up my very irritable injury. Charlie combines this wealth of knowledge with a great rapport and easy-going energy.

I went from walking at a snail's pace, to running and playing volleyball in three weeks. He set me up for prevention of future injuries and gave me tools to use on a daily basis that are easy to work into my schedule and gave me instant results. I would recommend a friend or family member with a spine injury to Charlie and would definitely return in the future, if needed."

– Jen Sosnowski, DPT

" I came to see Charlie because of a constant ache in the thoracic area of my back. He immediately was able to diagnose the problem, showed me exercises I could do at home, and did physical therapy manipulations on my back (e.g. to loosen up the stiff joints to get the blood flowing) that made all the difference. I no longer have the constant ache in my back. Charlie is a consummate professional, cares deeply about his clients' success and cares deeply about what he is doing. I highly recommend him!"

– L.M.

" I came to Charlie for my lower/mid back pain, I was immediately impressed that Charlie listened and didn't just start recommending treatment plans without first knowing my symptoms and issues. In the past I had a Physical Therapist recommend exercises that actually made my pain and issues worse and did not listen at all. I was by no means a text book case, but Charlie took the time to find out what worked for me. He would try exercises and then adjusted them for what worked best for me.

I would highly recommend Charlie for any of your physical therapy needs. He is friendly, educated and most importantly listens to your concerns to make sure you are comfortable while still challenging you. I was very pleased with my treatment provided by him."

– Chantel Orcutt

Now, I want you to know that this book is a quick and dirty guide to lower back pain and sciatica...designed to help you get fast, effective relief in the comfort of your own home (or wherever you may be reading this).

By NO means is this meant to fully replace specialized, in-person advice and care from a trained professional.

Keep in mind, the tips and tricks that you will read in this book will not only provide relief and increase your awareness of how you do day-to-day things, but they are 100% backed by science and experience.

As I mentioned to you earlier... I traveled coast to coast and searched high and low for how to best treat people just like you...

In fact, here's a picture of me with the road trip crew before we left for California.

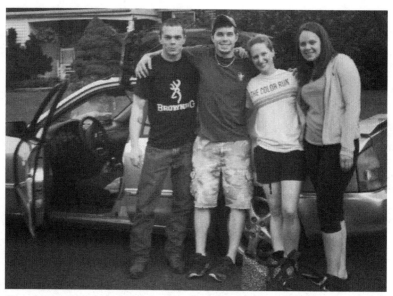

(from left to right) My younger brother Brandon, me, my loving wife Heather, and her cousin Stephanie.

Oh yeah, I graduated with my Doctorate of Physical Therapy from Lebanon Valley College (a small private college in Central Pennsylvania), practiced for some time, and then realized I was addicted to learning to better help other people.

So... I applied for the University of Southern California Orthopedic Residency Program, the #1 rated physical therapy program in the country... and eventually accepted a position to work and teach at the University.

Pretty neat, right!?

During my time there, I worked side-by-side a top-notch spinal surgeon and learned a ton about lower back pain and sciatica that I'll share with you in this book.

Here's a picture of me and the homeward bound crew again the night before the roadtrip back east...

It's at my white coat ceremony (graduation) as I finished at USC...

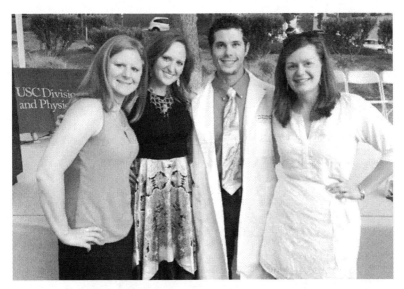

(from left to right) My sister-in-law Shannon, my biggest fan and wife Heather, me, and my partner in crime during PT school & best friend Erika"

I'm back on the east coast now and I've written this book to help people just like you who are looking for answers and hoping for relief without the use of drugs, injections, or even worse...surgery.

Now, all these insider secrets would mean absolutely nothing if you didn't start using them ASAP.

The single biggest mistake people make when they have lower back pain is they ignore it.

Realize that most lower back pain and sciatica starts off as a "stiff back" that just feels overworked...

BUT, as you ignore what was once only causing some lower back stiffness, you may begin to irritate nerves in your back causing leg pain, numbness or tingling.

Scary, isn't it?

OK... not really... it doesn't have to be scary at all. Because as you'll learn later in this book... the body has an amazing ability to heal itself... it was designed to move, lift, and twist.

But it can cause you to worry and wonder what is causing such weird feelings.

Because of this, I do urge you to take action fast.

As with any problem, the sooner you get things taken care of... the better.

You will sleep a lot better (literally) if you get a jumpstart on things and start using the strategies in this book.

What are you waiting for? Relief is just pages away...

Happy Reading,

Charlie Johnson, PT, DPT, OCS

PS – If you have any questions as you go through this book, you can email me directly at **charliejohnsondpt@gmail.com** and I'll get back to you.

Chapter 1

Getting To Know Your Back

The most important piece of your recovery is that you understand all you can about what is causing your pain and problems.

This is true for every part of life...

Once you have identified a problem, you must understand what the problem is, how it got there, and what options you have to fix it.

You are likely to experience quicker relief of your symptoms if you take the time to read and understand the following information.

First things first, here are some quick facts about the spine...

The spine is made of a stack of bones called vertebrae. There are 33 vertebrae in total and there are 5 main regions in the spine...

1. The cervical spine (or neck), which includes 7 vertebrae.
2. The thoracic spine (or mid-back), which includes 12 vertebrae.
3. The lumbar spine (or lower back), which includes 5 vertebrae.
4. The sacrum, which includes 5 vertebrae formed together.
5. The coccyx (or tailbone), which includes 4 small vertebrae formed together.

Between most of the vertebrae are discs, which act as spacers and help absorb shock. The bones and discs in the lower back are the largest in the spine.

Picture the discs in your back as mini jelly donuts. On the inside of the discs, there is a jelly-like material made mostly of water (called the nucleus pulposus), and the outside of the disc is created by a wicker weave of layered tissue (called the annulus fibrosis) that helps form the shape of the disc and keep the jelly-like substance inside.

When two bones are stacked on top of each other, a joint is formed on either side... this happens at each level of the spine.

A spinal level is named by listing the number of the top vertebrae followed by the bottom vertebrae.

For example the L4/L5 spinal level would include the 4th and 5th bones in the back, as well as the disc between them.

Between each level in the spine is a pair of nerves (31 pairs of nerves in total) that branch off the spinal cord on each side and exit the spine through holes called intervertebral foramen.

Now, what are nerves?

Nerves are like highways.

They act as a 2-way path for information related to feeling and movement.

This information is constantly being sent up and down the pathways to tell your body what's going on around you and how you should act.

Healthy nerves allow us to feel and move in small or big ways depending upon the situation.

Think about the tiny ant you can feel crawling on your foot during a summertime picnic.

Think about the cool draft that you notice as someone opens the door on a winter night.

Now, think about when someone scares the living daylights out of you and you flinch at the speed of light.

Yup... all signs that your nerves are healthy and fully functioning.

Now that we know nerves are like highways carrying messages of feeling and movement, we must understand that nerves are real living structures within the body that move as you move.

Healthy nerves should be able to do 3 things:

1. **Glide** – Picture a game of tug of war. For example, as you pull your toes towards your nose, it pulls on the nerve from one end of your leg...but pull your knee towards your chest and it will pull on the nerves from the other end near your hip. Nerves are like long ropes that will move whichever way they are pulled.

2. **Compress** – Have you sat in a funky position only to find that your foot falls asleep? This is the result of nerve compression. Shake it out and your feeling comes back.

3. **Tension** – Using the idea of tug of war, picture a game where strength from both teams is equal and both are pulling with the same force on either end of the rope. This would result in tension of the rope or, for the purpose of this book, the nerve.

When a nerve loses its ability to glide, compress, or withstand tension because of an injury, poor posture, or overuse... it can become sensitive.

Sensitive nerves will often cause feelings of weakness, burning, shooting, numbness or tingling.

Simply put, there is a problem somewhere along the highway. In the lower back and leg, the sciatic nerve commonly becomes sensitive... when this happens, it is called sciatica.

Sciatica is numbness, tingling, burning or shooting that is felt down one or both legs in a narrow band that occurs when pressure is placed on a nerve.

The sciatic nerve is the largest nerve in the body, and is made up of 4 main spinal nerve roots that exit the spine...L4, L5, S1, S2 OR the 4th and 5th lower back nerves and the 1st and 2nd sacral nerves.

Remember, nerves are like HIGHWAYS...

Pinched nerves are like highways with traffic jams that cause temporary closure of some or all of the lanes.

If we close one of these lanes, we slow the sending of information and we end up with feelings of pain, weakness, numbness, or tingling.

(Keep reading to discover the 3 most common causes of lower back pain and sciatica...)

Just as you may take certain highways to get from one destination to another, nerves do the same.

Feeling and movement to different parts of the body are controlled by certain nerves.

As you learned above, there are 4 main nerves that make up the sciatic nerve...

L4, L5, S1, S2 OR the 4th and 5th lower back nerves and the 1st and 2nd sacral nerves.

Think of them as highway L4, L5, S1, S2.

Each of these main nerve roots provides the leg with a specific area of feeling. Look at the diagram below...

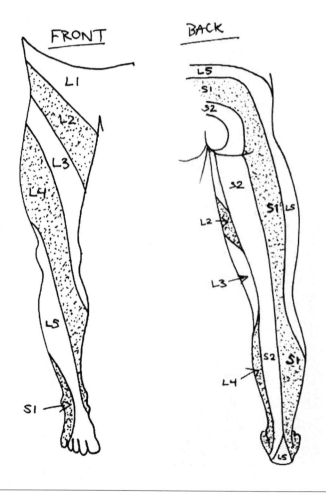

For example, the most common pinched nerve in the back is the L5 nerve (or the 5th nerve in the lower back).

So, people with this problem often feel pain in their buttock, which runs to the outside of the knee, and then wraps around the front of their shin towards their big toe.

Now, it's not always that clear-cut, but by looking at this diagram you might be able to tell which nerve could be causing you an issue...

Final thought - the feelings you may have from a pinched nerve are only temporary. They heal naturally with time, gentle exercise, and specialized treatment.

Chapter 2

The 3 Most Common Causes of Lower Back Pain and Sciatica

#1 Herniated Disc

The single most common cause of lower back pain and sciatica is a Herniated Disc.

What Is a Herniated Disc?

A herniated disc, also known as a bulging or slipped disc, occurs when the inner jelly is pushed outwards through a tear in the outer portion of the disc resulting in a bulge or herniation (kind of like when jelly is squeezed out of a donut). They can happen in any part of the spine, but are most common in the lower back.

A herniated disc can cause dull, achy pain in the back, buttock, or leg... and if large enough, may even press on nerves in the spine causing sciatica.

What Is Sciatica?

Sciatica is numbness, tingling, burning or shooting that is felt down one or both legs in a narrow band that occurs when pressure is placed on a nerve.

What Does Sciatica Feel Like?

The most common feelings are pain, numbness, and tingling in a narrow band down the leg. Everyone is unique though... here are some common ways people may describe feelings from sciatica:

- Electric
- Burning
- Weakness
- Shocking
- Coolness
- Bee Stings
- Shooting
- Trickling Water

One lady even told me, "It feels like ants are crawling on me..."

Point being... sciatica can create many unusual and scary feelings...

Good thing is... sciatica goes away.

What Causes a Herniated Disc?

Herniated discs can occur from excessive strain or injury, or degeneration due to age. When the pressure on the disc is too much for the outer portion of the disc to handle, a tear may occur, which allows for inner jelly to bulge or herniate outwards.

So Where Does The Herniation Usually Occur?

In most cases, the bulge occurs at the back of the disc and to one side. Behind the disc lies a nerve on either side of the spine.

Pain is usually felt in the central part of the lower back, but leg pain, numbness or tingling due to pressure on a nerve is usually only felt on the side of the bulge. The most common level of a herniated disc is L4/L5 - which may put pressure on the L5 nerve (the 5th spinal nerve in the lower back). In severe cases, the inner jelly may actually leak outside of the disc or put pressure on the bundle of nerves at the base of the spinal cord.

10 Telltale Signs of a Herniated Disc

1. Pain that "Comes & Goes"

If your lower back pain is due to a herniated disc, your back tends to "go out" on you once or twice a year. When it does, you often have lower back pain that makes it difficult to stand up straight. If severe, you may notice pain, numbness, or tingling down the leg.

2. Central Lower Back Pain

Herniated discs usually cause pain slightly above the belt line that remains in the center of the back or spans across the lower back from one side to the other.

3. Sciatica

The most common cause of sciatica is a herniated disc.

4. Pain with Sitting

As we sit, we place pressure on the front of the disc, which causes the jelly-like material in the disc to be pushed backwards. This places pressure on the outer part of the injured disc and sometimes the nerves in the spine.

5. Pain When Going from Sitting to Standing

Lower back pain due to a herniated disc causes stiffness when getting out of a chair or out of the car after sitting for a while.

6. Pain with Coughing & Sneezing

Coughing and sneezing increases pressure on the discs. When a disc is herniated, excess pressure on the discs caused by coughing and sneezing may be painful.

7. Less Pain Standing

When we stand, we take pressure off the front of the disc and place pressure on the back part of the disc, which helps push the jelly-like material in the disc to be pushed forwards away from the injury and away from the nerves.

8. More Pain Bending, Lifting or Twisting

When we bend or lift or twist, we increase the pressure in our discs. People with herniated discs often notice lower back pain when they bend, lift, or twist in an awkward position.

9. Pain is Worse in the Morning

Pressure within the discs of the lower back are highest in the morning after a restful night sleep. When we first get up in the morning, we compress the spine again, causing a sudden increase in disc pressure... which can cause pain if you have a disc herniation.

10. Whole Body "Shifted" to One Side

If you've ever "thrown your back out" or had it "go out on you," you may notice that it's very hard or painful to stand up straight. You may feel crooked or notice yourself leaning to one direction if you look in the mirror. Often the body tilts away from the side of the disc herniation to avoid compressing the painful area. This is a strong sign that a disc herniation is likely causing your lower back pain.

Can Disc Herniations Heal?
Yes, herniated discs become smaller by reabsorption as healing cells help remove injured disc material. Most disc herniations heal within 3-6 months, letting you get back to a normal, healthy life.

What should I do to help heal herniated discs and prevent them from happening in the future?
You should know that it's common for back pain to "re-occur"... and this is normal, but follow the tips below to give yourself the best chance of staying pain free.

• Sit up tall by using a back support when in a chair or while driving.

• Lift with your legs, not your back.

• Take frequent breaks if doing activities that require you to be bent over for an extended amount of time... every few hours, place your hands on your hips and arch your back 10 times.

• When you lift, get close to the object you are lifting and keep the object close to your body when you carry it (the further the object is away from your body when you lift, the more pressure you'll place on your back).

• Sleeping on your side or your back is best for the discs.

#2 Spinal Stenosis

What is Lower Back Spinal Stenosis?

Spinal stenosis is narrowing of the spaces in your spine, which causes pressure on the spinal cord or nerves that travel from the spine into your legs.

What Causes Spinal Stenosis?

Stenosis is most commonly caused by disc degeneration and/or arthritis in the lower back, which causes the spaces in your spine to narrow... giving less space for your spinal cord and the nerves in your back to travel. Spinal stenosis causes sciatica in one or both legs depending on where the nerves are compressed.

What Are The Types of Spinal Stenosis and What Do They Feel Like?

In order to best understand the two types of spinal stenosis, think of the spine and the nerves in the spine as a tree with branches. Using this example, it will be easy to understand the two main types of spinal stenosis and why you may be feeling what you're feeling.

To help you understand this, I'd like you to walk through a simple activity. Start by grabbing a piece of paper and a pencil...

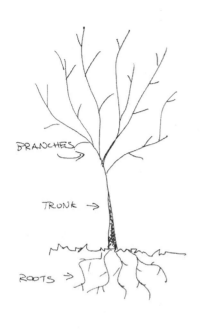

BRANCHES

TRUNK →

ROOTS →

Step 1:

Draw a tree...roots, branches and all. Like this...

Now, imagine it's a nice spring day and you're cleaning up your property by cutting down some trees.

You decide to cut the first tree at the trunk of the tree... naturally, the entire tree above where you cut falls over.

The next tree you decide to only cut a branch off. Only the branch that you cut off is gone, the rest of the tree is alive and well.

Make sense?

Cool.

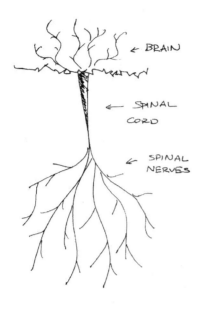

BRAIN

SPINAL CORD

SPINAL NERVES

<u>Step 2:</u>
Flip your paper so that the tree is upside down. It should look something like this.

This should start to remind you of the spine...

To help orient you, think of the roots as the brain, the main trunk as the spinal cord, and the many branches on either side as the spinal nerves.

Applying the concept above, we can understand the two types of spinal stenosis and why you feel what you feel.

The first type is Central Spinal Stenosis: Narrowing of the central canal of the spine where the spinal cord travels... which causes lower back pain and leg pain, numbness, and tingling in both legs.

This could be likened to you cutting the tree at the trunk. In this type of spinal stenosis, the main spinal cord (or trunk) becomes compressed... which causes problems for everything below this level. This is why leg pain, numbness, and tingling is felt in both legs.

The second type is Foraminal or Lateral Stenosis: Narrowing of the holes (intervertebral foramen) where the nerves exit the spine... which causes lower back pain and leg pain, numbness, and tingling in one leg.

This could be likened to you cutting just a single branch off the tree. In this type of spinal stenosis, only one spinal nerve or branch is a problem...the rest of the nerves, including the main spinal cord (trunk) is fine. This is why pain leg pain, numbness, and tingling is felt only in one leg.

5 Telltale Signs of Spinal Stenosis

1. Older than 50 Years Old

People with spinal stenosis as a result of disc degeneration and/or arthritis in the spine are generally older.

2. Leg Pain is Worse than Back Pain

Pain with spinal stenosis causes compression of the nerves in the spine called neurogenic claudication. This often causes leg pain that is worse than lower back pain.

3. Leg Pain, Numbness, Tingling with Walking/Standing

When we walk and stand, our spine is upright, which causes the spaces in the back where the nerves travel to narrow. This causes compression of these nerves, which results in pain, numbness, or tingling.

4. NO Pain with Sitting

People with spinal stenosis usually sit to relieve their pain. In fact, they often have no lower back pain or sciatica when they are sitting. When we sit, we bend the spine forward, which opens the spaces in the spine and relieves compression on the nerves by giving them more room to travel.

5. "Shopping Cart Sign"

Pain from spinal stenosis is often relieved by leaning forward while walking. Have you ever seen a person leaning forward on a shopping cart while at the grocery store? If so, we call this a "Shopping Cart Sign." These people may be trying to relieve pain from spinal stenosis. Remember, when people with stenosis lean forward, there is less pressure on the nerves, which helps relieve pain, numbness, tingling in the legs that occurs with walking/standing.

Can Spinal Stenosis Be Helped?

While the aging process of the spine cannot be reversed, people with spinal stenosis can learn specific exercises and day-to-day tips to help relieve their pain. The goal of these exercises is to help relieve pressure on the spine and nerves.

Generally, people with spinal stenosis respond best to exercises that involve bending the spine forward, with the goal of relieving pressure on the spine and nerves...

Sitting in a chair with your legs apart, reach down towards the floor slowly as if placing your palms flat on the floor.

When you've reached the floor, hold this position for 10 seconds. Do this 10 times every few hours throughout the day.

Eye-Opening Fact:

Recent research shows only a small relationship between the amount of spinal stenosis and arthritis in the lower back found on an X-ray and the pain that you feel. Many people have spinal stenosis and don't even know it.

#3 SI Joint

What Is The SI Joint and Where Is It Located?

There are actually two SI Joints, one located on either side of the tailbone. Each SI Joint is formed by the connection between the tailbone and the pelvic bones.

What Is The Purpose Of The SI Joint?

The SI Joint is a stress relieving joint that helps absorb shock from above and below. When bending, lifting, and twisting, forces from the lower back travel into the pelvis... When walking, going up/down stairs, or running, forces travel up through the legs and into the pelvis. The SI Joint helps transfer forces and absorbs shock as we move throughout the day.

How Common Is SI Joint Pain?

15-30% of people with lower back pain have pain coming from the SI Joint.

Who Gets SI Joint Pain?

SI Joint pain occurs across the lifespan. In general, 3 groups of people may experience SI Joint pain:

1. Young & Active People

When we are young, our lower back bones and pelvis are still very flexible - sometimes too flexible. If the SI Joint moves too much, it can cause pain.

2. During and/or After Pregnancy

During pregnancy, hormones are released to help relax the pelvis to prepare for childbirth.

These hormones hang around for some time after pregnancy, which results in the pelvis becoming more flexible. Again, this can cause pain/problems.

3. Older People After Lower Back Surgery

Remember, the SI Joint is a stress relieving joint. After surgery, the lower back may not move as well as it had before surgery... this causes your body to try and move elsewhere. Sometimes this can cause extra stress on the SI Joint.

4 Telltale Signs of SI Joint Pain

1. Pain Below the Level of the Belt Line on One Side

The SI Joint is located below the level of the belt line within the pelvis. Problems here cause pain below the belt on one side of the tailbone. While SI Joint pain can rarely cause two-sided pain, people with SI Joint problems most often have one-sided pain due to a one-sided pelvic problem.

2. Pain When Going from Sitting to Standing

Remembering that the SI Joint helps transfer forces as we move... lower back pain due to the SI Joint often causes pain when moving from one position to the next.

3. Pain Rolling Over in Bed, Climbing Stairs, or Standing on One Leg

Movements that cause the pelvis to be uneven may stress the SI Joint.

4. Pinpoint Pain

SI Joint problems often make a very specific region in the pelvis sore to the touch at the location of the SI Joints on either side of the tailbone.

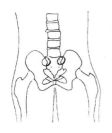

Remember, SI Joint pain is usually one-sided. The picture to the left is a view of the lower back and pelvis as if looking from the back to the front. Circled is the area of pinpoint pain that most people with SI Joint problems feel.

What Should I Do to Help Relieve SI Joint Pain?

- Avoid crossing your legs when sitting.

- When sleeping on your side, place a pillow between your knees to keep one leg from crossing over the other while you sleep.

- Limit exercises that are high impact or where your weight is not evenly distributed (this would include things like jumping, running, or lunges).

So, I'd be lying if I told you that finding the cause of your lower back pain and sciatica and then treating it was always easy. While I couldn't possibly cover every cause of lower back pain and sciatica in this book, the above 3 (alone or in some combination) are the most common.

Chapter 3

What's Going On? Self-Movement Tests You Can Do At Home

In this chapter, I will review specific self-movement tests to help you better determine the cause of your lower back pain and/or sciatica. By now, you understand the telltale signs of the 3 common causes of lower back pain and sciatica. After reading these, you may already have a good idea of what could be causing your pain.

Follow along with the following self-movement tests to better determine the cause of your lower back pain and sciatica.

Herniated Disc and Sciatica:

Remember, the #1 cause of sciatica is a herniated disc. If you've read through the telltale signs for herniated disc and you are beginning to believe that you have sciatica...try these self-movement tests at home.

Here are two self-movement tests to determine if you have sciatica:

#1. Slump Test:

How It's Done: Seated on the edge of a chair or bed, slouch your whole body forward so that your back is rounded. Bring your chin slowly towards your chest, as if looking down.

Next, pull your toes and ankle up, then slowly attempt to straighten your knee.

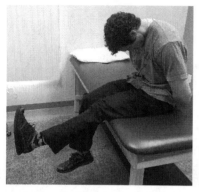 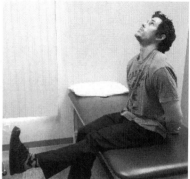

As soon as you feel your pain...stay in that position for a moment, but keep the entire position the same and only lift your head up (as if looking up towards the ceiling).

What It Feels Like: If you have sciatica, you will notice that it is more difficult and painful to straighten the leg of the side where you have your pain, numbness, or tingling. It may even cause pain, numbness, or tingling to travel down your leg...AND when you lift your head, your leg pain lessens.

A positive test would be if attempting to straighten your knee in this "slump" position causes pain, numbness, or tingling to travel down your leg...AND when you lift your head, your leg pain lessens.

#2. Straight Leg Raise:

How It's Done: Lying on your back, pull your toes and ankle up and slowly raise your leg towards the ceiling.

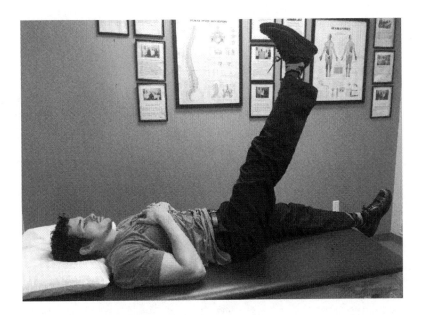

<u>What It Feels Like:</u> If you have sciatica, you will notice that it is more difficult and painful to straighten the leg of the side where you have your pain, numbness, or tingling. It may even cause pain, numbness, or tingling to travel down your leg.

So...a positive test would be if you feel pain, numbness, or tingling when attempting to perform the straight leg raise.

You may also notice that raising the opposite leg of where you feel your leg pain (the pain-free leg) causes an increase in your lower back pain. If this happens, it is a very strong sign that your lower back pain and sciatica is due to a herniated disc.

These two self-movement tests gradually tension the sciatic nerve that runs from the back down the back of the leg to the foot.

Remember that healthy nerves have the ability to glide, compress, and tension without pain. If the sciatic nerve is sensitive, these tests will reproduce your pain and be uncomfortable.

On to the 2nd most common cause of lower back pain and sciatica...

Spinal Stenosis and Sciatica:

If you recall after reading the telltale signs, the classic sign of spinal stenosis is leg pain more than back pain that comes on with walking or standing and goes away with sitting. The key in this is the position of the spine.

When we stand tall, we narrow the spaces where the nerves travel... creating less space for them to function – which causes leg pain, numbness, or tingling when up and about. When we bend our spine forward, as in sitting, we create more space for the nerves to travel and relieve pressure on them. Because of this, people with spinal stenosis very rarely feel leg pain when sitting or bent over.

Knowing this, I have designed a self-movement test for you to try. Here it is...

Shopping Cart Test:

How It's Done: Head out to your local grocery store and grab a cart. Start by walking upright as you push the cart. You may notice that your leg pain, numbness, or tingling begins after just a couple of minutes walking up tall.

When you notice this, stoop forwards as your push the cart, using the cart for balance...now, continue to walk like this.

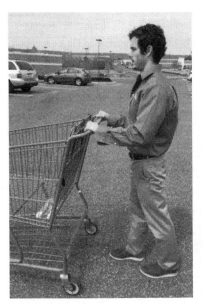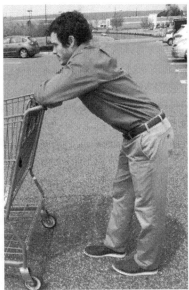

What It Feels Like: If you have spinal stenosis causing your leg pain, you may notice that pushing the cart while standing tall eventually increases your leg pain, numbness, or tingling. BUT when you stoop forward and continue to walk, the leg pain lessens and you are able to walk better. If you stand back up again, your leg pain will return. Stoop forward and it again lessens or may even go completely away... just like a light switch. On-Off-On-Off...

A positive test is when walking/standing upright brings on your leg and lower back pain, but stooping forward relieves it.

Now onto the third common cause of lower back pain...

SI Joint:

The SI Joint is a joint, and therefore, does not have the ability to cause numbness and tingling. If you feel numbness or tingling, you may still have an SI Joint problem, but it is usually not the main cause.

Again, if you've read through the telltale signs of SI Joint pain, then you should try out these two self-movement tests.

Remember, SI Joint pain is almost always one-sided and below the level of the belt line - without numbness or tingling.

#1. Thigh Push Test:

<u>How It's Done:</u> Lying on your back, take the leg on the painful side and bend it up to 90 degrees (as shown). Place your hands on top of the knee and attempt to push the thigh straight downwards towards the floor. Hold the push for 2 seconds, then release. Complete up to 5 times.

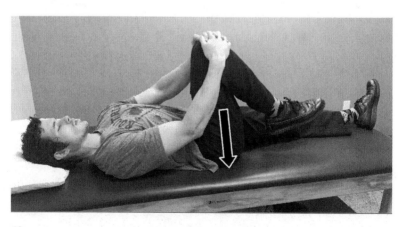

<u>What It Feels Like:</u> If you have SI Joint pain, you will likely feel a slight increase in your one-sided lower back pain when you push the thigh towards the floor.

A positive test is one that increases your one-sided lower back pain.

#2. One-Legged Bridge:

<u>How It's Done:</u> Lying on your back, straighten the leg on the pain-free side and bend the other one up. Keeping everything level, attempt to push into the floor and lift your bottom off the ground as shown. Pause at the top for 2 seconds, then lower yourself down. Complete up to 5 times.

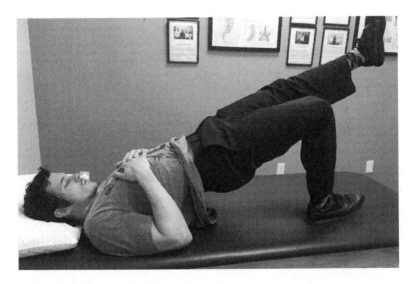

<u>What It Feels Like:</u> If you have SI Joint pain, you will likely feel an increase in your one-sided lower back pain when you lift the hips off the floor.

A positive test is one that increases your one-sided lower back pain.

There you have it...

Self-movement tests to better help you determine the cause of your lower back pain and/or sciatica. But remember, everything should make sense.

You should have most of the telltale signs on top of positive self-movement tests in order to feel sure about what could be causing your pain.

Read on to discover my top 3 exercises for each of the common causes of lower back pain and sciatica...

If you've read through the telltale signs and performed the self-movement tests and you're still not sure what could be causing your lower back pain, numbness or tingling... I'd love to hear your story. Email me directly at **charliejohnsondpt@gmail.com** if you're looking for help.

Chapter 4

Top 3 Exercises for Herniated Disc, Spinal Stenosis & SI Joint

Below you will find my top 3 exercises designed specifically to help you find relief from a herniated disc, spinal stenosis, or SI Joint pain. Up to this point, the puzzle of what could be causing your lower back pain or sciatica should hopefully be clearer. The telltale signs should match what you feel and are experiencing, as well as the results of the self-movement tests.

Using what you know now about the 3 common causes of lower back pain and/or sciatica, follow the step-by-step instructions to perform my top 3 exercises for what you feel could be causing your pain.

Herniated Disc

#1. Back Arches

How It's Done: Lying on your belly, place your hands flat, just above the level of your shoulders. Keeping your hips on the table, press your upper body towards the ceiling, as if doing a push-up. Hold 2 seconds at the top, slowly lower and repeat 10 times every 2 hours.

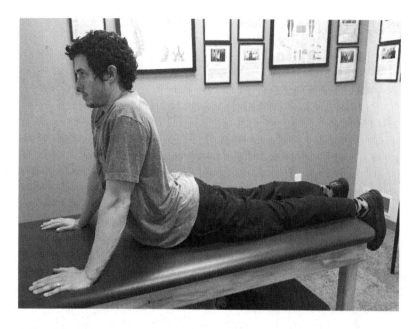

<u>Why It Works:</u> It helps gently move the lower back and relieve pressure.

#2. Up Tall Straighten Leg

<u>How It's Done:</u> Sit up tall on the edge of a chair or bed until you feel slight tension in your lower back. Slowly straighten your leg to the point just before you feel your pelvis tip backwards or your back round- then pause for one second. Slowly lower and repeat 20 times each leg. The goal is to keep the back tall throughout the entire exercise. In fact, it doesn't matter how much you straighten the leg- all that matters is that you keep the back straight and up tall. If you straighten the leg and the pelvis rocks backwards, you've gone too far.

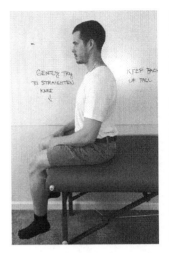 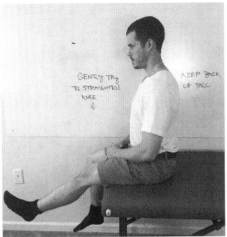

<u>Why It Works:</u> It strengthens your lower back and teaches you to control the way it moves.

#3. All Fours Rocking Back

<u>How It's Done:</u> On your hands and knees (on the floor or bed), let your lower back and spine gently fall towards the floor until you feel a slight arch in your lower back. Slowly rock backwards keeping this lower back position. Pause when/if you reach a point in the motion where your lower back begins to round. Return to the starting position and repeat 20 times. The goal is to keep the back tall throughout the entire exercise. Again, it doesn't matter how far you rock back- all that matters is that you keep the back straight. If your back rounds, then you've gone too far.

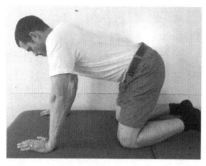
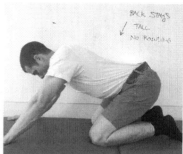

<u>Why It Works:</u> It strengthens your lower back and teaches you to control the way it moves.

Spinal Stenosis

#1. Trunk Twists

<u>How It's Done:</u> Lying on your back, knees bent up and feet flat on the floor, let your hips and legs gently twist side-to-side. Pause when you feel a stretch on either side for 2 seconds. Repeat 30 times each direction. (This one works well first thing in the morning)

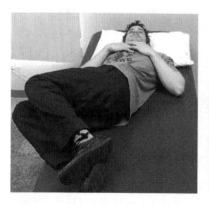
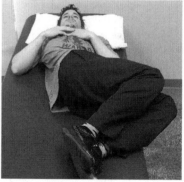

<u>Why It Works:</u> It helps to restore pain-free motion in your lower back in order to lessen your stiffness and make you feel looser.

#2a. Seated Bend

<u>How It's Done:</u> Seated on the edge of a chair, legs shoulder width apart, gently reach towards the floor until a stretch is felt in your lower back. Hold stretch for 10 seconds and then return to sitting upright. Repeat 10 times.

Do this exercise 3-5 times throughout the day.

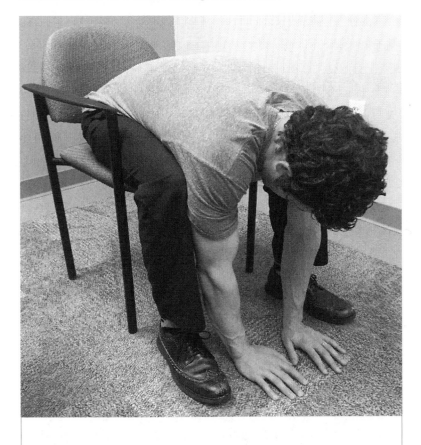

 IMPORTANT: If you have been diagnosed with osteoporosis or "brittle bones," then avoid this one, but do this instead...

#2b. Knees to Chest

How It's Done: Lying on your back, gently pull both knees towards your chest until a stretch is felt in your lower back, hold 10 seconds 10 times. Do this exercise 3-5 times throughout the day.

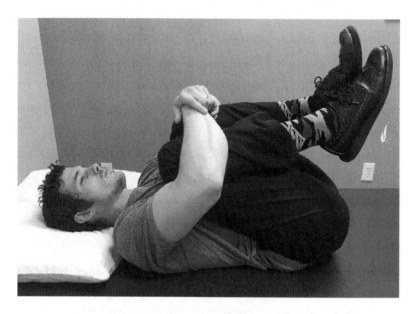

Why It Works: These exercises help increase the spaces where the nerves travel, which helps to relieve pressure on the nerves.

#3. Standing Pelvic Tilt

How It's Done: Standing with your back against the wall, feet about 1 foot from the base of the wall, tighten your belly muscles as if raising your belly button. You should feel your pelvis tilt backwards and your lower back flatten against the wall. Hold 10 seconds 10 times.

Hint: Once you get the hang of this...try holding this position as you walk by keeping your belly tight. You may notice that it reduces your lower back pain as you walk.

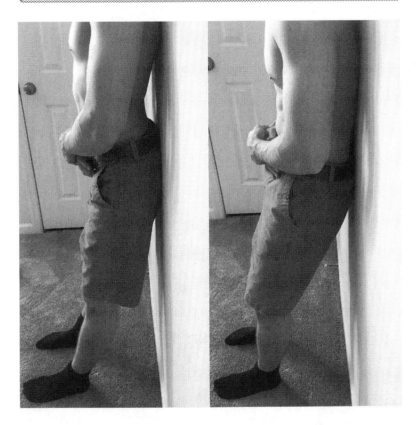

Why It Works: This exercise helps increase the spaces where the nerves travel, which helps to relieve pressure on the nerves. It also "turns on" the muscles in the belly, which allows for the muscles in your lower back to relax.

SI Joint

#1. Clamshell Holds

How It's Done: Find an old belt and buckle it. Lying on your side, keeping your feet together on the ground...place the belt around your knees and press outwards against the band as if trying to open your legs. Keeping moderate pressure against the band, hold for 60 seconds. Repeat 3 times. No cheating... stay on your side, no rocking backwards. (Then flip over and repeat on the other side.)

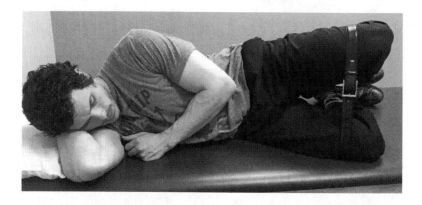

Why It Works: You'll feel this exercise working in the deep hip muscles, which help stabilize the pelvis and the SI Joint.

#2. Bridge Holds

How It's Done: Lying on your back, place the belt around your knees and press outwards against the band as if trying to open your legs. Keep your feet on the ground; they should be shoulder width apart. Keeping moderate pressure against the band, lift your hips into the air and hold 30 seconds. Repeat 3 times.

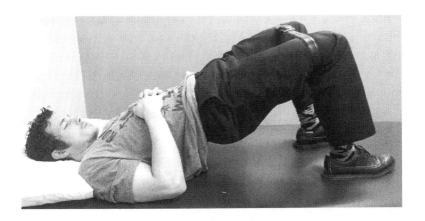

<u>Why It Works:</u> Pushing outwards activates the deep hip muscles. Lifting your hips towards the ceiling activates the buttock muscles, which help stabilize the SI Joint.

#3 Squat Holds

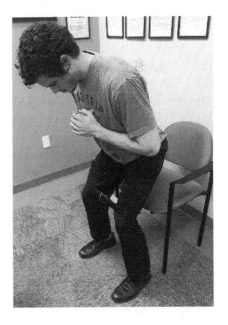

<u>How It's Done:</u> Sitting in a chair, with your belt around knees, feet shoulder width apart, push outwards against the band with moderate pressure. Keeping pressure against the band, stand up slowly from the chair, pause at the top 1 second still keeping pressure outwards against the band. Sit back down (pressure still against band). Do 20 sit-stands.

<u>Why It Works:</u> Often people with SI Joint problems have pain going from a sitting to standing position. By placing pressure outwards against the belt while you go from sitting to standing, you'll better activate the hip muscles and stabilize the pelvis.

Chapter 5

Getting In Touch With Your Pain

Okay...soooo...up to this point, you've learned a ton about lower back pain and sciatica.

If you followed along step-by-step, you've also reviewed many telltale signs of lower back pain and moved on through your very own self-movement tests.

Now that you're pretty sure what could be causing your lower back pain and sciatica, it's time to dig a little bit deeper. What do I mean? Well... I want to teach you how to "get in touch with your pain" using several strategies that I use every day with the people I treat.

The purpose of the following activities is to help you really understand your pain and help you figure out how to control it.

That's right you heard it.... I'd like to teach you how to control your pain.

This is super important.

What I've seen over the years is that the feeling of having no control over the pain is what really freaks people out and keeps them from getting better.

You've already done half the battle if you understand that you likely have full control over the pain caused by your lower back and can make it better or worse just by the way you do every day activities.

You see, people who go through the exercises below can learn how to gain full control over their pain.

Would you be surprised if I told you that the people who believe they will get better are the ones who actually do get better?

Surprise or not - it's the truth.

Remember, lower back pain and sciatica doesn't last forever...chances are you have the power to grab a hold of your pain and change how you feel today.

Now, enough is enough...put some serious thought into these exercises below and I'll walk you through each one step-by-step.

Step One: Where do you hurt? What do you feel and how much do you hurt?

Using the body diagram below, mark where you hurt using the symbols to describe what you feel and where you feel it.

Be specific – just a pain in the back or down the back of the leg? Is the numbness and tingling in the whole leg or just the outer side?

The more specific, the better.

After marking down where it hurts and what it feels like, write how much it hurts. Using a scale of 0 to 10...where zero equals no pain and 10 equals the worst imaginable.

Go ahead and mark it down.

Going even a step further...write down your pain level right now, at its worst, and at its best.

Sharp Pain	Achiness	Burning	Pins & Needles	Numbness
////	XXX	!!!!	OOOO	++++

Instructions: rate your major area of pain on the 0-10 Pain Rating Scale below:

0	1	2	3	4	5	6	7	8	9	10
No pain		Weak	Moderate		Strong		Very Strong			Maximal Pain

Please rate your pain (0-10) at rest and with activity in the spaces provided:

With Activity _____   **At Rest** _____

Ok great...now onto Step Two.

Step Two: Finding out what makes it better and what makes it feel worse by creating what I call a "Trouble Tree."

Step One helps you put your feelings on paper so you can "see what you're feeling..."

But, now let's learn why you might be feeling what you're feeling by identifying your aggs and eases...that is those things that aggravate or make your symptoms worse and those things that ease your pain or make you feel better.

This is where you really start to feel a sense of control.

For this exercise, grab any blank piece of paper (a piece of copier paper works just fine).

At the top of the page, write "Trouble Tree."

Below that, but still the top of the page, write your name followed by "lower back pain"...then circle it.

It might feel weird writing that...or maybe even a little scary...but now you own your pain and when you own it and understand how to control it, you can make it go away for good.

All right, this is where some serious brain power will be needed...

I need you to think long and hard about the things you do in everyday life that increase your symptoms. You know – things that increase your lower back and sciatica and make you feel worse.

If you haven't thought of any just yet, I find it helpful to start by working step-by-step through your day; hour-by-hour from the time you get up to the time you go to sleep–big picture things, such as sleeping, driving, computer work, typing, reading, watching TV, and sitting.

List these activities by drawing lines from your center bubble branching outwards.

It should start to look like a tree...a Trouble Tree.

Now that you've got some main activities that increase your pain, use the other half of the page to think about what decreases or eases your pain.

Same idea, create a separate branch for each and put a bubble around it.

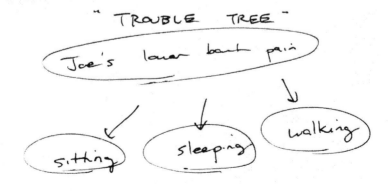

Soooo...the purpose of this exercise is to give you a BIG picture viewpoint of what makes you feel better and worse.

While creating the Trouble Tree, you'll also become more aware of how you're feeling, which will be super helpful to understand when healing.

Think of healing like a big see-saw.

In order to get control your pain and problems, you have to find the right balance of activities that make you feel better and those that make you feel worse.

In other words:

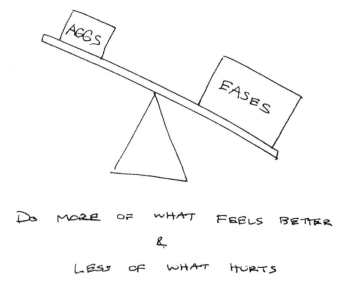

Do MORE OF WHAT FEELS BETTER
&
LESS OF WHAT HURTS

If you can learn to do more of what makes you feel better and less of what makes you feel worse, you almost always win...meaning the power to get a hold of your pain is unlimited.

For each aggravating factor, get more specific and create more detailed branches.

For example, if sitting bothers you, it could look like this:

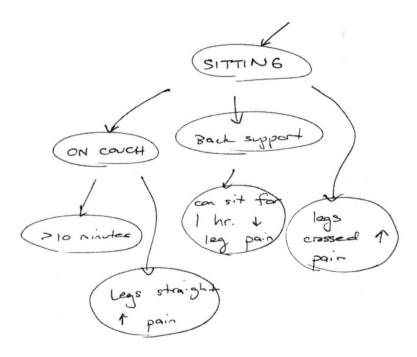

OR if walking bothers you...

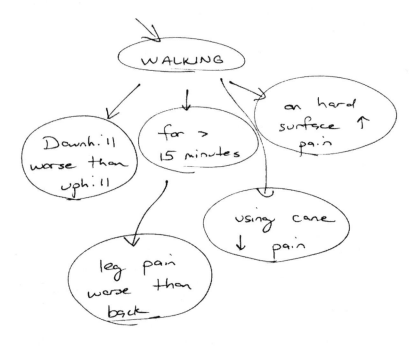

You may start to notice a trend...

By getting to the nitty-gritty of what really bothers you, you can start to change the way you do these things.

After you've worked through each aggravating activity and you've thought long and hard about what activities are bothering you, it's time to start doing things differently (I'll give you more tips in the upcoming chapters).

But remember the equation - if you're not sure how to change what makes things worse, do more of what makes you feel better.

Start doing more of what relieves your pain and less of what makes it worse.

Step Three: Journaling

Step Two is tough, but it's key in giving you control of your pain and showing you the big picture of how you feel.

If you're stumped and feel like the last step didn't go smoothly, give journaling a try...

Grab a notebook and start documenting what you're feeling.

The key things to document include: the date, time, what you're feeling, what you were doing when you felt it, how long it lasted, and what you did to make it go away.

We could create columns or just include all these things in each entry.

Carry a little notebook around with you...bring it to work, sit it by your nightstand, bring it wherever you go for 1 week to track your symptoms.

Often you may start to see a pattern.

Then, go back and fill in your Trouble Tree blanks using what you've learned through journaling.

Here's an example of a journal from an actual patient of mine:

Journal

3/12/16   7:32pm
Sitting on couch
 — legs straight = pain increased
 into left calf. Bending knee =
 calf pain decreased. Sitting
 "up tall" = increased lower
 back pain, but decreased
 leg pain.

3/13/16   6:15am
sleeping
 — laying on right side increased
 left leg pain. But pillows
 under right side decreased
 leg pain.

After doing this activity, you should feel more in touch with your pain and better understand what you can do to relieve your pain...which allows your body to heal.

Although this may sound strange, I want you to feel more "in touch with your pain"...BUT I don't want you to feel worried about your pain.

In fact, pain is a good thing. Pain is your alarm system.

Let's talk about it...

Chapter 6

All About Pain

Warning! This chapter may fire you up, make you feel confused, or change your life...

No matter what happens, it's a must read.

The information I include below is a summary of research performed by some of the gurus in understanding pain (Lorimer Moseley, David Butler, and Adriaan Louw...see the citations at the end of the book if you're interested in learning more).

Pain is normal.

Pain is an experience created by the brain to protect you from threatening situations and injury.

Even if no problems exist in your body, nerves, or immune system... you may still feel pain if the brain thinks you are in danger.

Simply put, without your brain, you feel no pain.

Think of your brain and the pain you experience as your alarm system...

In everyday life, you have a "normal" threshold for pain - as your nerves buzz around happily waiting to react to whatever your body feels.

So your alarm system is set and ready to go.

In normal everyday life, your alarm system looks something like this:

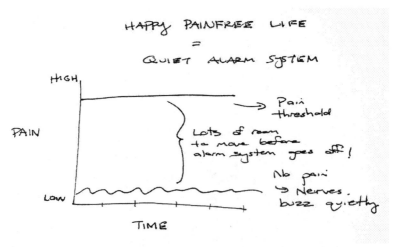

Now, if you hit your finger with a hammer, it would look something like this:

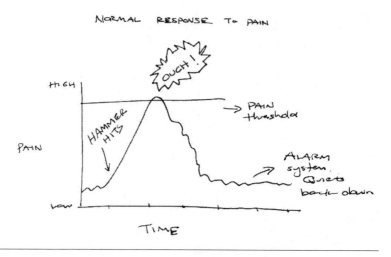

It hurts like heck, but eventually after several hours/days, it calms down to where it was before.

Now, imagine you've had lower back pain for a long time...it's likely that your alarm system has become extra sensitive and now it looks something like this:

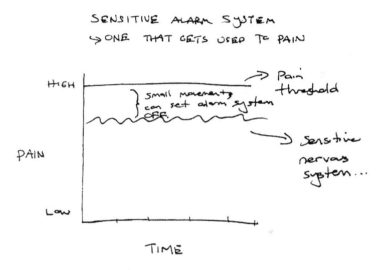

If it's not making sense, think of it like this...

It leaves little room for you to do things before your alarm system goes off.

When we are not in pain and life is grand, it takes a lot for your alarm system to go off – just like a car's alarm when you have to break the windows in order to set the alarm off.

Now, when your body's been in pain for some time, the alarm system becomes extra sensitive – Instead of having to break and bash the windows before the alarm goes off, a leaf blower goes by and your alarm goes berserk!

Simply put... your body's alarm system becomes sensitive and leaves little room to move and do things without feeling pain.

Important Point: Pain does not equal damage or injury...it is simply an experience created by the brain when it thinks your body is in danger.

Imagine you get a paper cut...

Wouldn't you be worried if the pain stuck around for months?

Sure you would, because normally the pain goes away in minutes to hours.

Then what makes your back any different?

Most people live with lower back pain for years...yet this simply couldn't be caused by a simple injury to your lower back muscles or disc.

Why?

All tissues in your body heal, including the muscles, ligaments, discs and nerves in your lower back within about 3-6 months.

When pain lasts longer than 3-6 months or becomes chronic and lasts for years, it doesn't mean that something is wrong with your back or your back didn't heal properly, it simply means that your alarm system is sensitive...and for some reason, your brain still senses danger.

Think about when you get a bruise and are not aware of it...

As long as your brain doesn't sense danger, you won't feel pain.

Another Point: You're not crazy...pain is very real.

BUT remember, pain is an experience...

We've all heard about the crazy stories of people who are injured and feel absolutely no pain.

Picture the soldier injured in war who continues to run in order to save his life.

OR the man who had his arm trapped in between two rocks and cut his own arm off in order to escape the wilderness and survive. Yikes... but a true story.

On a more basic, less extreme level...think about the pain someone would feel if they hurt their back while running across a busy highway versus getting out of a chair.

I'd be willing to bet that the person running across the highway feels much less pain than the person who's getting out of the chair.

So, situation can impact pain.

Other things that can change your pain experience include emotions, beliefs, sleep, your job, or your pain memories... just to mention a few.

Emotions: People who feel sad or worried often feel more pain. People who are happy and relaxed generally feel less pain.

Beliefs: Growing up, some people were taught to be afraid of pain or that pain is bad. Others were taught to "get up and brush it off." Depending on your beliefs about pain you may feel more or less pain.

Sleep: People with good sleep habits generally feel less pain. I recommend 8 hours of sleep per night. Restful sleep has been shown to decrease the sensitivity of your alarm system.

Job: People who have stressful jobs and are unhappy with their careers often experience more pain compared to those who enjoy their work.

Memories: If your back was injured in a car accident...just thinking about driving could make your pain worse. Pain memories can be powerful.

Now, you should be asking yourself, "How do I calm my alarm system down?"

First things first, in order to calm your alarm system down, we need to review a few key points:

Point Number 1: Understand that pain does not equal harm.

Just because you feel pain doesn't mean anything serious is wrong... it just means you're alive and your alarm system is on high alert, that's all! Your back heals itself in 3-6 months, but your alarm system might still be sensitive.

Point Number 2: Pain does not equal gain. Remember, even though pain is created by the brain, which can sometimes cause your alarm system to become extra sensitive...even when everything has healed, it is very real. And you should still listen to it.

Okay, now that you understand these two big points, here's how you can begin decreasing the pain that you experience...

Respect pain and listen to it, but do not fear it.

Again, pain is normal...sometimes the brain gets a little confused and senses pain incorrectly.

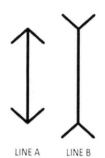

Take, for example, the two lines here... Which line is longer?

Pretty clear that it looks like line B is longer than line A, right?

LINE A   LINE B   But actually, they are exactly the same length.

Sometimes the brain can do the same thing when it comes to pain... it senses pain incorrectly OR it thinks there is actually something dangerous when really everything is just fine.

Gentle movement and exercise helps relieve pain and release chemicals that soothe nerves and calm down your alarm system.

Choose a form of exercise you enjoy...walking, biking, or swimming are all great options.

Slowly increase the amount of time you exercise week by week. Exercise up until the point you start to experience your pain, then stop. If you stick with it, you should notice that you are able to do a bit more week by week with less pain.

Okay, so this is really going to make you think...

Recent research has clearly shown that there is little to no relationship between the issues found on an X-ray or MRI and the pain you feel in your lower back.

That is to say, just as many people with pain have bulging discs as those who have absolutely no pain at all.

The same goes for spinal stenosis. (More on this later...)

Wrapping things up here...

- Understanding your pain will be super helpful in getting back to normal and living a healthy, pain-free life.

- Pain is normal and is caused by so much more than just injury... it is an experience that can be made better or worse by many things in life.

- Even though pain is created by the brain, it is still very real, and is our body's way of protecting us.

- Sometimes our brain can become confused and cause us to feel pain even after our body is healed...in other words, our body's alarm system becomes extra sensitive.

- By understanding pain, changing the way you think about pain, and regularly exercising...you begin to reset your alarm system and your pain experience.

Chapter 7

Day-2-Day Strategies

You should be in touch with your pain by this point and should better understand what things make your pain better and worse.

You should also understand how pain works and may even be feeling "at ease" already.

Now, I'll share with you some of the day-to-day activities that many people struggle with when they have lower back pain and sciatica.

In other words, I'll discuss some common activities that make things worse...then I'll show you how to change these activities to make things more tolerable.

But, I'll warn you...all of these tips demand change.

Here we go...

1. Sitting

Think about the shape of your back when you sit. Often, our spine forms a "C" shape as we slouch forward in our chairs at work. Sometimes, this can cause extra pressure on the structures in your lower back.

To change the way you sit, follow these simple steps below:

Step #1 - Sit Up Tall
This is the simplest tip, but often the most difficult habit to break.

Nothing else matters if you can't sit up tall.

Oddly enough, we all know what this means... (In fact, you probably just did... keep that going)

Step #2 - Setup For Success
To combat a slouched posture, we must properly setup our seating environment.

If you sit at work all day, adjust your work environment to best fit your needs.

Use the tips below to help you have less back pain throughout the day.

First, stop reaching and pull your chair in...back against the chair.

Reach in all directions...get a sense of your reach zone.

Now, move all commonly used items within your reach zone (phone, important documents, stapler, post its, calculator, pen, etc.).

If driving, sit up tall and pull your seat closer. This will cause your knee to bend more, which can sometimes relieve pressure on sensitive nerves.

Step #3 – Stay Grounded

Before I go into detail here, I have a brief experiment for you...

Sitting up tall, feet on the ground...get a sense of the position of your spine.

Ask yourself three questions – Does it feel arched? Rounded? OR feel slouched?

Now, keeping those questions in mind...cross your legs.

What happens?

Chances are, your pelvis rocks back, your lower back rounds, and you slouch forward.

All of the above strategies won't matter much if your feet aren't flat on the ground (and by this I mean no crossing your legs).

A healthy position is a position where you remain grounded...
Lower your chair so that you can reach the floor or use a stool to place your feet on.

Step #4 – Get Some Support

In Step 2, we discussed the importance of keeping your back against the backrest of your work chair. You will soon realize that without knowing it, you fall back into old habits.

No worries, this step will help you prevent this...

Use a lower back support.

You may feel as though your chair is supportive enough...and if so, skip to the next step, but I still recommend you give it a try.

Here is how you make one at home using nothing more than an old towel, duct tape, and a belt or string.

There are two methods that you could try - pick whichever feels most comfy.

Option One: Back Support

Follow the order of the pictures to properly make a lower back support. (When finished, the roll should be 4-5 inches thick.)

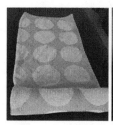 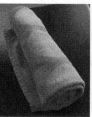 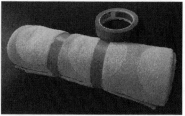

Step 1: *Take a large bath towel or beach towel and fold in half.*   **Step 2:** *Tightly roll.*   **Step 3:** *Tape the roll together to keep it from coming undone.*

> **BONUS TIP:** Feed a belt or rope through the center of the towel, so you can attach it to a seat and keep it from moving.

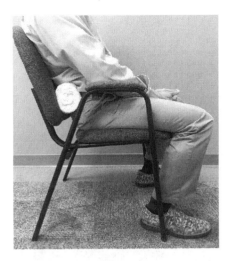

Place the towel roll behind your back like this... right about the level of the belt line. This will help keep your back up tall when you're sitting.

Option Two: Buttock Role...

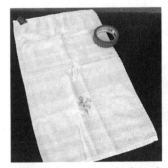

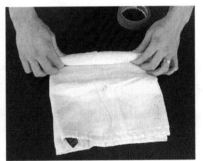

Step 1: *Take a medium sized towel.*   **Step 2:** *Tightly roll it up.*

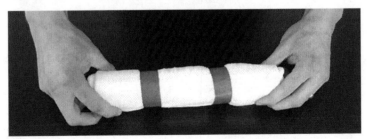

Step 3: *Tape the roll together to keep it from coming undone.*

Now, placement ... don't make this mistake...

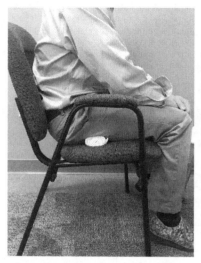 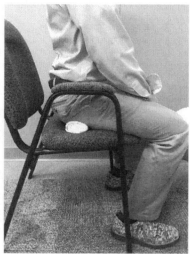

Under the buttock...you should NOT be slouched back like this (the roll is likely placed too far forward).

Instead, you should be sitting up tall, like this...

So you now have two options of how to put your back in a better position. It's amazing how just changing the position of your pelvis can put your lower back in a better position.

Step #5 – Stay Active

Get up from your chair every 15 minutes to keep your spine and muscles loose.

Also, start a walking program at home or on lunch breaks at work to get the blood flowing and prevent things from stiffening up.

2. Sleeping

I could write a whole book on sleeping...

One of the biggest problems for people with lower back pain and sciatica is that they have a difficult time finding a comfy position.

In order to sleep better, you first need to understand sleep PATTERNS and POSITIONING.

Not only does sleep affect the way you feel, but it alters how well your body functions.

The amount of sleep that one gets has been directly related to the pain one feels.

Less sleep = more pain the brain senses.

That's right...remember, pain is perceived in the brain and people perceive pain differently.

Okay, let's talk about Sleeping Patterns.

Simply put, commit to one and stick to it.

Find a time that is reasonable for you to go to bed each night that will allow you at least 8 hours of sleep.

That's right, 8 hours... sounds crazy, but it's not too bad (if you wake at 6am, plan to be asleep by 10pm).

AND as an added tip: close the iPad, put down your smartphone, and shut down the TV...it's well known that looking at these bright screens just before shut-eye can keep you from falling asleep.

Now on to Sleeping Position...

Usually, the best sleeping position for people with lower back pain and sciatica is on the back.

Now, while some of it is personal preference, I've found that most people prefer firm sleeping surfaces. Some people even tell me that they have less leg pain when they sleep on the bare floor.

If you find it difficult to sleep on your back, give these modifications a try...

1. Sleep with a towel roll under your back

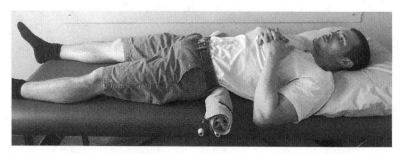

2. Pillows under your knees

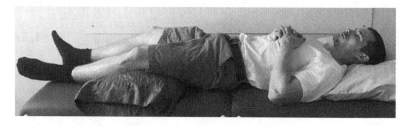

The next best position is on your side. Give these positions a try to help relieve your lower back pain or sciatica...

1. Pillow between your knees

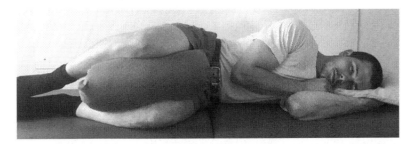

2. Pillow under your side (if you have one-sided lower back or leg pain, it usually feels best to lay on the pain free side with a pillow underneath)

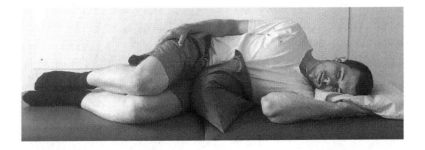

Lastly, lying on your belly is considered to be the least friendly for your lower back.

But, in all honesty, if it helps...do it.

3. Bending and Lifting

Bending and lifting is something that many people with lower back pain are careful of, avoid, or are afraid to do because of how it makes their lower back feel.

Often, this is how people injure their lower back.

There are two big factors that determine how much pressure you place on your back when lifting.

1. Position of the Back

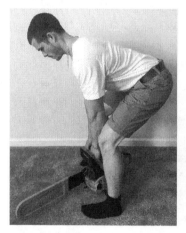 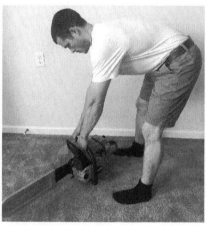

When lifting, keep your back straight like this.

Here's what's NOT to do...

2. Distance of the Object from the Body

When bending down or lifting, keep the object you are bending towards as close to the body as possible. The further the object is away from you, the heavier it feels.

4. Walking

While it is difficult to change the position of your spine when you walk, I do have a couple suggestions if things are really bothering you...

- In the worst case scenario, use a cane or walker to decrease your leg pain, numbness, or tingling when you walk. Hold the cane on the side opposite to the leg that hurts. This will help reduce the pressure on your back and leg.

- When shopping use a shopping cart...You've likely figured this one out by now, or seen others doing it, but by leaning forward on a shopping cart it can temporarily relieve the pressure on your lower back.

- Take frequent rest breaks to avoid setting off your alarm system and increasing your pain.

- Refer to the Top Exercises for Spinal Stenosis: Try the final exercise...the Standing Pelvic Tilt exercise against the wall. Once you get the hang of it try keeping a similar position when you walk. Do this by thinking about "keeping your belly tight." By doing this, you will shift your body weight backwards, which will activate the muscles in the front of the belly and shut off the muscles in your lower back. Simply put, it changes the way you move and what your lower back feels. See the pictures on the next page to better understand how your muscles work when you move.

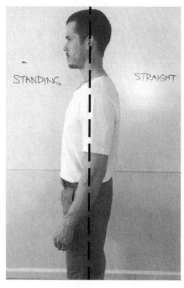

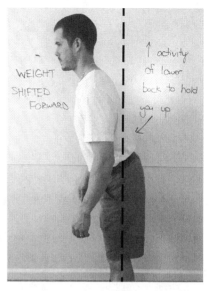

1. Normal Standing:
Equal balance between the front abdominal muscles and lower back muscles to keep you standing.

2. Standing with back arched and forward lean: *Increased use of lower back muscles to keep you from falling forwards. This position often increases pain in people with spinal stenosis.*

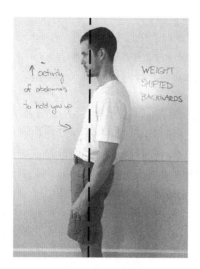

3. Standing with belly tight, pelvis tilted backwards and slight backwards sway: *Decreased use of lower back muscles and increased use of abdominals to keep you from falling backwards. In this position, the back is NOT arched, the belly is kept tight and the weight is shifted slightly backwards. This position often decreases pain in people with spinal stenosis. Now...I've exaggerated the position here, but the basic concept is to keep the belly tight while walking to prevent your back from arching and lower back muscles from working overtime.*

Those are the 3 most common activities that bother people with lower back pain and sciatica. By trying to change the things that make you feel worse, you can begin the healing process by doing less of what hurts and more of what makes you feel better.

Chapter 8

X-rays, MRI, and Nerve Testing: The Good, The Bad & The Ugly

There's a natural progression of lower back pain and sciatica that I see all the time. It usually goes something like this...

You gradually begin to feel lower back pain or stiffness for no reason... OR you bend, lift, twist and feel a "twinge" in your lower back.

A day or two later, the stiffness seems to be sticking around and "stretching it out" doesn't seem to be helping much.

You become more aware of your pain and your alarm system becomes more sensitive.

You begin to notice a dull ache in your buttock or back of your thigh.

What used to be just lower back pain begins to turn into occasional leg pain, numbness and tingling that travels down the back of the leg towards the foot.

You become concerned and realize that you need some help...

You pay a visit to your family physician and here's what they say:

"Well... You definitely irritated your back and you might even have a pinched nerve. Here...take some of these (anti-inflammatories and muscle relaxants) they should help. Come back in two weeks if it doesn't feel any better. Then, I'll send you to get an X-ray."

Now, one month after this all began, and a couple doctor visits later, you get an X-ray that shows arthritis in your lower back, a bulging disc or two, and decreased space between the bones in your back due to degenerative disc disease (DDD for short).

Perhaps your physician even recommended physical therapy...this is a great start.

OK STOP...let me explain.

The first step any physician will take when trying to determine the cause of your lower back pain is to order an X-ray.

1. X-ray

What Is An X-ray?
X-rays are relatively inexpensive images to take pictures of the bones in your body (in this case, usually the back and pelvis) - you can't see muscles, ligaments or nerves...only bones.

The Good:

- They're low cost.

- They make sure you have no fractures or bone disease that could be causing your pain.

The Bad:

- X-rays will find everything and anything that is wrong with the bones in your back and pelvis. Unfortunately, these "problems" on the X-rays may not be causing your lower back pain or sciatica.

- Exposure to radiation.

The Truth:

There is little association between things found in your back during an X-ray and what you actually feel.

50% of people with absolutely no lower back pain or sciatica have arthritis, bulging discs, and degenerative disc disease.

These findings are often completely normal - like wrinkles on our skin as we age.

Now, you've had an X-ray and may even be going to physical therapy to try and relieve your lower back pain and sciatica, but you still aren't feeling much better.

You likely have lower back pain and leg pain, numbness, tingling or weakness.

The second step would be to get an MRI...

2. MRI

What Is An MRI?

An MRI is a test that takes pictures of the soft tissues of your body, including the muscles, ligaments and nerve pathways.

Like X-rays, they can also look at bones with great detail.

They take photos in slices so that you can look layer by layer through the back and spine to see what could be causing your lower back pain and sciatica.

MRIs pick up things like bulging discs that can press on nerves.

The Good:

- Very detailed imaging that lets you look layer by layer through the spine to see what could be causing your pain.

- No exposure to radiation.

The Bad:
- Expensive.

The Truth:

Recent studies show that people who have had an MRI and know the results heal slower than those who do not have an MRI.

Why? Again, imaging is great and all...but remember, just because they find something on an MRI doesn't always mean it's the cause of your problem.

Getting an MRI and being told you have many problems in your lower back makes people more worried about their lower back pain, rather than remaining calm and staying active.

Simply being told you have a bulging disc can make your alarm system more sensitive.

Okay, so you've had stubborn lower back pain and sciatica that is also causing your foot to drag or making it difficult for you to rise up on your toes...

The next type of testing is nerve testing...

3. Nerve Testing

What Is Nerve Testing?
Nerve testing includes two different tests:

EMG (Electromyography) – the use of small needles to assess the function of individual muscles in your lower back and legs (looking for abnormal muscle activity).

NCV (Nerve Conduction Velocity Testing) – Uses a device that provides small electrical currents to your nerves to test how quickly the signals are flowing down the nerves.

Together, they look for problems with how the nerves function and try to find a level in your lower back where the nerve might be having an issue.

The Good:
- Best tests to determine the health of the nerve.
- Used in combination with an MRI to determine the level of the nerve problem.

The Bad:
- Expensive.
- Often painful and uncomfortable.
- Results and accuracy are only as good as the person doing the test (I've found that there are very few people who do these tests well).
- Won't always find a nerve problem (even if you really do have one) if your pain started within the past few weeks. It takes time for nerve problems to show up on these tests.

X-rays, MRIs, and nerve tests are the most common tests used to determine the cause of your lower back pain and sciatica.

While they each are used for a specific reason, the results mean very little if a good clinical test is not performed.

Think back to your physician visit...did they have you touch your toes, arch your back, twist side-to-side, check your reflexes and try to get to the root cause of your problem?

Or did they just give you some pills and send you for an X-ray?

Anyways, understand that these tests aren't perfect by any means and should always be compared to what is found during clinical testing by a skilled healthcare provider, such as a physical therapist.

Also, don't let common results of arthritis, bone spurs, degenerative disc disease, herniated disc, or pinched nerves freak you out...

These findings are common in many people who have absolutely no pain at all.

One of the most common questions I hear when people come to physical therapy is...

"I have arthritis... can physical therapy help with that?...
There's nothing you can do to change my arthritis, is there?"

Here's my answer...

"Great question, while I can't do anything to physically change the arthritis in your lower back...there are many things we can do to improve how your lower back moves and the muscles in your back work. Also, you might find it interesting to hear that many people with arthritis have absolutely no pain at all. Recent research is actually showing little connection between what is found on an X-ray or MRI and the pain that people feel. Let me use a quick analogy to help you better understand how it's possible for people with such "ugly" things like arthritis and degenerative disc disease on an X-ray or MRI can have absolutely no pain.

Here's the analogy that I learned a while back... "Pain is like the wind." Think about it...

Can you see wind? No

Can you feel wind? Yes

Now, you can "see" that it's windy by looking at the environment around you, but that's merely a result of your past experiences and what you understand about how wind works and feels. You might see a flag or papers blowing, or someone's hair swaying back and forth...these things tell you it's windy.

I can't hand you a cup of wind, right? Because you've already agreed that you really can't "see" wind, you can only feel it...you should also understand that you can't take a picture of it.

All you can take a picture of is how it affects the environment around it...a "windy" environment.

The same goes for pain, pain is a feeling...not something you can see.

Therefore, a picture cannot be taken of pain.

Pain is an experience created by the brain to protect you from danger.

Just because an image shows arthritis doesn't mean you will feel pain...remember pain is not a thing that you can "see"...it's a feeling.

This is why people with arthritis in their lower back often have no pain at all.

That's not to say that the arthritis isn't there or that you aren't feeling pain, it just means that, luckily for you, it doesn't have to cause you an issue.

In fact, it's super common in almost everyone. Make sense?

A floor that is swept might look clean and shiny at first glance, but under a microscope, you'd be sure to find all kinds of things...sort of like an X-ray or MRI.

If you look hard enough, you are likely to find something.

In people that are pain free and have "healthy" backs, X-rays and MRI are sure to find everything and anything that could be going on.

Okay, so, that being said...while I can't change your arthritis, I'll look at the way you move and listen to what's going on and come up with a plan to help you. Likely the plan will include some form of hands-on physical therapy to make you move better and decrease the sensitivity of your lower back as well as exercises to help get you moving better."

There you have it...my fully exposed reason for why what is found on an image may not be what's actually causing your pain.

Sounds crazy, I know...but it's absolutely the truth.

This is why people with "bad backs" on X-ray or MRI may feel nothing at all.

Bringing things full circle...and back to the natural timeline of how lower back pain and sciatica develops...know that the quicker you get treatment the better.

The longer your alarm system is sensitive, the harder things can be to calm down.

X-rays and MRIs are great for making sure nothing "big and ugly" is going on (such as a fracture or tumor), but less helpful for common things such as arthritis, disc degeneration, or herniated discs that are found in most people.

Chapter 9

The Truth About Medications, Injections and Surgery

This book wouldn't be complete without talking to you about what other treatments are available to decrease your lower back pain and sciatica.

You may have asked yourself already... What if the strategies in this book don't help me or what if physical therapy doesn't work?

The order of treatment from least invasive to most invasive goes as follows:

Physical Therapy > Medications > Injections > Surgery

I'll start off by saying that good hands-on physical therapy works for many people.

I'll also say, sometimes you might need a little extra help to recover by using medication, getting an injection or in rare cases... needing surgery.

The first line of defense in the treatment of any lower back pain is (or should be) physical therapy ---which offers a completely natural treatment to get the joints in the lower back to move better, muscles firing and relieve pressure on the nerves.

Often times, physicians will prescribe medications to help decrease the inflammation in the lower back and nerves and many times they can be very helpful in the short-term. Medications include anti-inflammatories, pain relievers, and/or steroids. But taking any medication long-term can be bad for your health.

According to research, anti-inflammatories are among the most commonly used medications. It is estimated that they cause over 100,000 hospitalizations and result in 16,000 deaths per year because of the intestinal damage they can cause. Yikes!

Anyways, anti-inflammatories including Advil, Motrin, Ibuprofen, and Naproxen are one way to decrease pain and inflammation in the lower back. Another more powerful way is to use a steroid.

Steroids are usually taken over the course of a week or two in a tapered fashion—where on day one you take a certain amount and then each day following you gradually decrease the dose.

Tylenol is a pain reliever and fever reducer. It is not an anti-inflammatory.

Also, take note that these medications are taken by mouth, so they don't just impact your lower back, they affect the whole body.

This leads me smoothly into the next line of defense... injections.

So, maybe physical therapy is "helping some" and drugs are working "okay," but you just haven't found a ton of relief yet.

Injections are likely the next step.

Injections to your lower back help relieve pain and inflammation because they are able to be aimed right at the spot of joint/nerve inflammation.

Injections are more specific than taking a pill by mouth and allow the medication to get closer to the root cause of your pain.

Surgeons use live imaging that allows them to see where they are placing the needle during the injection.

They inject the steroid, combined with a numbing agent, into the spinal canal, where the solution flows upwards through the spinal canal with the goal of soothing the joints and nerves.

Now, injections don't help everyone. About 2 out of 3 people get relief from an injection.

> **Warning:** If you have diabetes, be prepared that your surgeon might tell you they can't give you an injection because they often cause blood sugar to spike.

Finally...the last straw...

If you are going to physical therapy, taking medication, went and had an injection and still no relief...surgery is your last option...and I mean it should be your very last resort.

There are really 3 major types of lower back surgery to relieve lower back pain and sciatica:

1. Microdiscectomy

A lower back microdiscectomy surgery is performed to remove the portion of a herniated disc that is irritating a nerve in the lower back. A microdiscectomy is performed through a small incision in the lower back. A microdiscectomy may be needed if you begin to lose feeling or strength in the leg due to nerve compression.

The Truth: Data from research suggests that patients who have herniated discs have similar long-term outcomes whether they undergo surgery or choose conservative treatment like physical therapy.

2. Laminectomy

A laminectomy surgery is used to remove the back part of the vertebrae that covers your spinal canal. It is often used for people with spinal stenosis who have pain in their legs when they stand or walk due to pressure on the nerves in the lower back. A laminectomy enlarges your spinal canal to relieve pressure on the nerves (think of it as removing the roof on a house). It works like this...

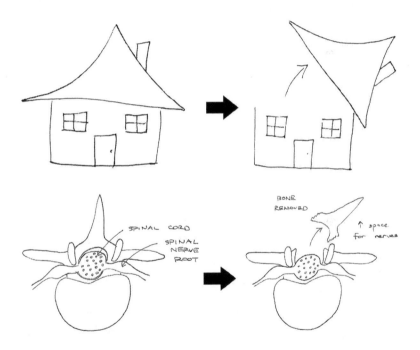

[Above] You're looking at a single vertebrae from a bird's-eye view, as if it was taken from your back... This drawing shows how removing part of the bone (laminectomy) creates more space for the nerves in the lower back.

3. Spinal Fusion

A spinal fusion is a surgery performed to hold or "fuse" two or more bones in the spine together so that there is no movement between them. It can be performed alone or in combination with the above surgeries.

Again while I've seen successful surgeries...they have the worst potential side effects of any other type of treatment that we discussed so far.

That being said, surgery is needed in some bad cases to prevent nerve damage.

Zooming out...medications, injections or surgery all have their place in the treatment of lower back pain and sciatica, but remember, they all have side effects.

Physical therapy is your best bet if you're looking for 100% all-natural relief.

Chapter 10

The 7 Must-Ask Questions Before Choosing a Physical Therapist

I've included this special chapter to help you carry out your very own behind-the-scenes investigation of physical therapists (or other healthcare providers for that matter) in your area.

In this chapter, you will discover the top 7 must-ask questions (with answers) that you should ask before choosing a physical therapist... they will help you make a better, more informed decision about the care you can expect to receive.

After all, you should be skeptical of who provides your care and choosing a PT is no different.

In fact, your choice of a PT could mean the difference between you getting back to doing what you love OR feeling stuck with little to no results.

Your choice...but if you love life as much as I do, I hope your health is a #1 priority.

Your physician might try to choose or recommend a PT for you, but I wouldn't just take their word for it. (That would be like buying a new car without first taking it for a test drive...)

I don't know about you, but I prefer to buckle up and take the wheel before putting my health in someone else's hands.

It's for this reason that I recommend you call and ask these critical questions before choosing your physical therapist.

Here are the 7 must-ask questions before choosing a physical therapist:

1. How Long Does My Treatment Last?

Answer You Hope to Hear: "You can expect your treatment session to last about 45 minutes to an hour."

Why It Matters: 45 minutes to hour long treatment sessions are just right. Not only does it allow time for you to receive hands-on treatment and exercise, but it also allows you the time to ask questions and get answers about your problem.

Understanding what's going on, why it's happening, and how to prevent it from getting worse are key things you should know.

2. How Much Time Will I Spend With My Physical Therapist?

Answer You Hope to Hear: "The whole time... from the moment you walk in the door to the moment you leave, your PT will be showing you the ropes and helping you get back on track."

Why It Matters: First, it's your health and you deserve good care. If the problem would have just gone away or taking painkillers really solved your problem or you could handle it on your own... then you wouldn't be on the hunt for a physical therapist.

Second, you're paying for it - unless you have some form of super insurance - you're paying good money to be seen by a physical therapist. Be wary of a PT clinic who tells you that you'll be there for an hour, but then tells you the PT spends 15 to 20 minutes with you. Where'd they go for the other 45 minutes? This brings me to question #3...

3. How Many People Does The Physical Therapist Treat Per Hour?

<u>Answer You Hope to Hear:</u> "Our therapists are dedicated to making you happy and healthy, so we treat only one patient per hour. You get their attention the whole time."

<u>Why It Matters:</u> You shouldn't settle for anything less than a physical therapist who delivers 100% focused attention for 100% of the time. What you will likely hear is "our therapists treat two to three patients per hour."

You'll quickly discover that if you asked questions 1 & 2, what they're really saying is, "your appointment will last about an hour, but your PT is required to treat multiple patients per hour, which means they spend about 15 to 20 minutes with you."

I've worked at PT clinics where I was required to see 6-8 patients per hour...yikes.

This brings us back to the same question of where does the PT go for the other 45 minutes? And so I would ask that question as well...

The truth is, you'll likely be doing many exercises on your own or sitting on heat/ice while you wait your turn. While these sorts of things have their place, wouldn't you rather have one-on-one direct attention that you deserve and are paying your hard-earned money for?

Finally, understand that if you are treated for 15 minutes but stay for one hour, you're being charged for the entire one hour... not just the time spent directly with the therapist.

4. Who Will I Be Treated By?
(believe it or not, it's not always a licensed physical therapist...)

<u>Answer You Hope to Hear:</u> "You'll be treated only by a highly specialized Doctor of Physical Therapy."

<u>Why It Matters:</u> You pay for and expect to be seen by a licensed physical therapist. There should be no exception to this answer. What you may find is that you are seen only by a physical therapist, but they spend little time with you OR you'll be passed off to physical therapy assistants (PTA's), athletic trainers (ATC's), or physical therapy aides. ATC's require 4 to 5 years of education, PTA's require 2 years of education, and physical therapy aides require no specific education or training. You may not know, but physical therapists are now required to obtain their doctorate

For the best chance of recovery, I'd request to be seen by a PT only.

5. Are Any Of Your Physical Therapists Residency Trained?
<u>Answer You Hope to Hear:</u> "Absolutely yes, our therapists are highly specialized to offer the latest and greatest care possible."

<u>Why It Matters:</u> Less than 5% of the PTs in the entire country are residency trained. After receiving a doctorate in physical therapy, some physical therapists apply to and attend a residency program. During these programs, they become highly specialized from intensive training in a certain aspect of physical therapy.

6. On Average, How Often And For How Many Weeks Should I Expect To Be Treated?

<u>Answer You Hope to Hear:</u> "Well, it completely depends on your condition, but most people only require one or two visits per week for an average of 4-8 weeks before they get back to doing what they love."

<u>Why It Matters:</u> Most physical therapy clinics offer cookie-cutter approaches... and while it is nearly impossible to get a perfect clear-cut answer before being fully evaluated, you should expect to be seen for no more than 1-2 times weekly.

Unfortunately, you will likely hear that the average physical therapy clinic will expect to see you 3 times a week for 4-8 weeks.

3 times weekly is overkill...resulting in more time away from your family/work, more travel time, and more money out of your pocket.

Nowadays, PT clinics are under a lot of pressure to keep visits up and profit high. Rarely, if ever, do you need to be seen 3 times weekly.

7. Will I See The Same Physical Therapist Every Time?

<u>Answer You Hope to Hear:</u> "Yes, all patients are treated by the same PT each visit. You will not be passed between therapists during your care."

<u>Why It Matters:</u> You'll want to be sure you stick with the same therapist every treatment. Switching back-and-forth between therapists can cause confusion and leads to the "new" therapist having to re-check and get to know you before the treatment begins...leaving you with more chatting and less treatment.

The relationship you form with your physical therapist is super important.

There you have it... the 7 Must-Ask Questions Before Choosing A Physical Therapist.

When searching for a top-notch PT in your area...go one-by-one through these 7 must-ask questions.

To help, I've created a "Summary Sheet"... complete with the questions you should ask.

Do your research, pick up the phone, and get started.

Don't be afraid to share these questions with family or friends in need... there's nothing worse than jumping into a decision only to later say "I wish I would have known..."

Here's the summary sheet I've created...

SUMMARY SHEET

Name of PT Practice:

7 MUST-ASK QUESTIONS BEFORE
CHOOSING A PHYSICAL THERAPIST

....

1. How long does my treatment last?

2. How much time will I spend with my physical therapist?

3. How many people does the physical therapist treat per hour?

4. Who will I be treated by?

5. Are any of your physical therapists residency trained?

6. How often and for how many weeks should I expect to be treated?

7. Will I see the same physical therapist every time?

Other Notes:

If you need help or have other questions, call me directly at **(484) 552-3767** or send me an email at **charliejohnsondpt@gmail.com**.

Chapter 11

The Bullet-Proof Action Plan

What you should do RIGHT NOW!

1. Determine what's causing your lower back pain and sciatica by reading the telltale signs and by taking the self-movement tests at the beginning of this book.

2. Get in touch with your pain through creating your very own "Trouble Tree" and journaling what things make you feel better and what makes you feel worse.

3. Get started using strategies in this book. Try the exercises and change the way you do everyday things.

4. Reach out to someone who can help. Use the 7 Must Ask Questions Before Choosing A Physical Therapist guide to help you find a PT in your area who may be a good fit. The sooner the better.

5. Remember that even though we don't like it - pain is your body's alarm clock saying "Hey, listen up, something's going on over here"...alarm clocks don't go on forever...therefore, you don't have to be in pain forever.

About The Author

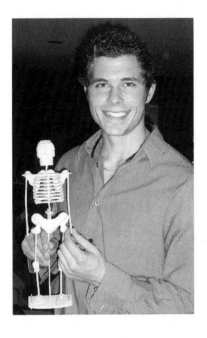

My Life Story, Why I Became a Physical Therapist, and My Unconditional Happiness Guarantee

I grew up in the small town of Schwenksville, PA.

Nothing really ever happened there, except for the yearly Chili Cook-Off at the Schwenksville Firehouse on Memorial Day and the Schwenksville Carnival in early June.

I met my wife there too...we went to Perkiomen Valley High School together and have been together ever since... "high school sweethearts" if you will.

Growing up, I was super active and played ice hockey...I was a goalie.

I loved exercising, eating healthy, and anything that involved me being outdoors.

In high school, I took an anatomy class and was interested in how the human body functioned and moved.

At the time, my passion for exercise combined with my newfound interest in the human body guided me towards a career in health and fitness.

While things were hopeful for me and I had a passion for health and fitness, I had a tough life growing up...and came from a very broken family.

At one point, as I applied to physical therapy schools, I ran into a major barrier...I had nobody to co-sign my loans.

Without a co-signer, I was essentially dead in the water and would be unable to pursue my passion.

Through my struggles in high school, I grew close to my high school guidance counselor...she really saw the best in me and was willing to do whatever it took to help me reach my goals. She offered to co-sign my loans that allowed me to get into PT school.

Pretty neat...and I was (and am still to this day) really grateful.

She had a huge impact on me.

Combining my love for exercise and the human body with my hopes of leaving a huge impact on people's lives (just like my counselor did for me), physical therapy was a natural fit.

After busting my behind through physical therapy school and graduating with my doctorate, I was ready to change the world.

I started working at an outpatient physical therapy clinic in southeastern PA.

Not long after starting, I knew it wasn't the right fit...

I became quickly frustrated by the lack of mentorship and enthusiasm, as well as the constant push to see more and more patients because of the control insurance companies had over the care of the people we were treating.

Within my first year, I had to make a major decision.

A large part of me was so turned-off by my profession that I considered quitting it all together.

Another part of me knew that I could do better.

As with anything in life, I knew that I would either "go big or go home"... And so I decided to apply to physical therapy residency programs.

These programs allow PTs to receive specialized training in a certain area of PT (like physicians who specialize in treating the heart – cardiologist, or the lungs or one who treats children – pediatrician).

Anyways, I got accepted... and traveled cross country to the University of Southern California, considered to be the "best-of-the-best" in all of physical therapy - #1 ranked PT school in the country.

On the west coast, I settled in to a new lifestyle. I was completely surrounded again by the environment I loved...one where people where always searching, asking questions, and striving to be the best.

However, the clinic that I worked in was again super busy, where I would see 4 or more patients per hour.

This made it difficult to practice in the best ways I knew how.

Armed with nothing more than a stack of books, my iPad, briefcase, and a burning desire to help people in the best way possible... I began planning to open my own private physical therapy practice.

And so now I have...

Here's the catch, my practice is completely out-of-network, and I don't foresee changing that anytime in the future.

This means I don't accept any form of insurance up front.

Doing so has allowed me the freedom to treat others like I would hope to be treated, with absolute 100% laser focused attention via one-on-one treatment sessions.

I've named my clinic "Physical Therapy & Johnson," because "Johnson PT" would be too generic... and well, there's nothing that bothers me more than "going with the flow" or "blending in."

The clinic is located in southeastern PA, not far from my hometown of Schwenksville, PA.

I've become dedicated to giving people world class care... so much so that I've created an "unconditional happiness guarantee" or your money back.

If you're not fully satisfied with the care you've received...

If you feel that you have not received the most in-depth, complete, and undivided care you've ever experienced... then you get your money back.

Now, some people think I'm crazy for offering this, and I guess in some ways I may be, but if you're anything like me, then health is your #1 priority... I truly believe that you deserve nothing less than the best care possible.

So, if you've read this book and are looking for help with your lower back pain and sciatica or you're interested in working one-on-one with me... I'd love to hear your story.

Feel free to reach out to me directly at **charliejohnsondpt@gmail.com**. I answer each email personally.

I hope you enjoyed this "Itty Bitty Book."

Happy Healing,

Charlie Johnson, PT, DPT, OCS
Physical Therapist
Board Certified Orthopedic Specialist
Physical Therapy & Johnson

PS – If you know someone else who could benefit from reading this too... send me a direct email at **charliejohnsondpt@gmail.com** with the subject line "Pay It Forward Book Request" and in the body of the email include their name, email, and address... I'll send one their way.

Success Stories

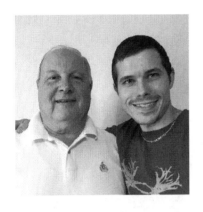

"I met Dr. Charlie Johnson in July, 2013, at a recommended Physical Therapy facility in the Pottstown, Pa. area. My Family Physician sent me for Therapy due to Sciatica Back Pain and Lower Back Disk issues. When I first met him I was in serious lower back pain and could not walk without assistance! At first visit it was quickly apparent Dr. Johnson was a Patient's Therapist! That means he focuses on curing the patient by first listening to why the patient has come for physical therapy and what do they have as "GOALS" at the completion of the doctor/patient therapy activity. After taking down the patient's dialogue on how they feel and what they want to accomplish, Dr. Johnson looks at the overall needs and physiological aspects of the patient's condition and only then prescribes a curative therapy path to follow.

In most cases he can forecast the timeframe involved to reach the patient's goals and a cure. While his approach may conflict with "Larger Therapy Businesses" that immediately begin with traditional therapy techniques and exercise routines, Dr. Charlie Johnson will ask Direct and Specific Questions that take him to the very best Physical Therapy techniques specifically needed by only that patient!

Today is July, 2016, and I have had no serious sciatica or lower back issues since completing my required "office" therapy sessions and "at home" exercise routines as of September, 2013. Dr. Charlie Johnson helped me walk again!"

– Bill Kopf

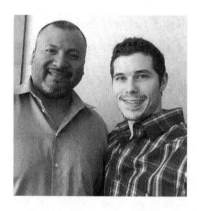

"On January 3rd, while playing with my son, I ruptured a disc on my lower vertebrate and landed in the hospital for 2 days. On January 6th, I stepped into the office of Dr. Charlie Johnson with the assistance of my wife, and a walker. I was 285lbs and compounding that with my back injury, I was in terrible pain. Painkillers were not helping as much as I've hoped. The pain, the injury, the weight, the lack of mobility and the thought that I would live with back pain for the rest of my life was just overwhelming. I came to Dr. Johnson with pain and not much hope. In fact, I believe one of my first questions that I asked Dr. Johnson after telling him my story was if I was going to be in pain for the rest of my life.

The answer that he gave me not only lifted my spirits, but ignited a fire in me to go and get better. He spoke to me about case after case of people that recovered from the same injury that I had and that although everyone was different, he didn't see a reason as to why I could not be part of the group that lived the rest of my life without pain.

This is how my journey began. I followed Dr. Johnson's advice. I did the exercises. I asked questions. And every time he would give me an answer, I would use that to fuel me past the pain. Every time I told him that I didn't want to do a particular exercise, he would just smile and tell me a different way to do the exercise to target the same muscle. With every visit, I would learn new things. From how to get out of bed (we went over this on my first visit), to how to put my socks on. And with every technique that he taught me, my ability to do things for myself just got better.

It was very difficult to get better. But here I am, almost two months later and I can honestly say that I'm a lucky person to have has Dr. Johnson see me and help me get better. I've lost 30lbs and changed my diet. I walk 3 to 4 miles per day. I do Yoga 2 times per week. And most importantly, I still do every single exercise Dr. Johnson recommended me to do every single day after every single one of my walks.

Thank you Dr. Johnson for showing a way to live my life that will help me continue my journey to a better "me"."

– Marvin S.

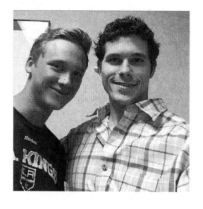

"I came in to see Dr. Charlie Johnson in the beginning of April with low back pain coming from a herniated disc. After seeing him over three visits I can probably say that I'm 98% better than I was when I started. Before I came in, the pain was so bad I could barely walk, now it barely hurts. Dr. Johnson is one of the best physical therapist that I've ever seen. Thanks for helping me get back on the mound."

– Joseph Risdall

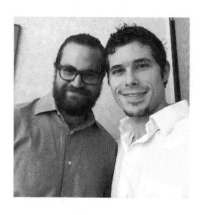

"Before I started working with Charlie, I was dealing with 2 straight months of excruciating Sciatica shooting down my left leg. I was unable to sit for more than a few minutes without major discomfort. Charlie right away showed me some corrective exercises that within a couple of weeks alleviated my pain and allowed me to recover much quicker from the pain. Months later, Charlie helped me to build a much stronger core, which will change my life forever. I'm grateful for all of his help through this experience and recommend him to anyone dealing with Back injuries!"

–Ayal Kleinman

Itty Bitty Disclaimer

All content found in this book was created for informational purposes only... to help you on your path to healing from lower back pain. The content in this book is not intended to be a substitute for professional, in-person, medical advice, diagnosis or treatment. It is impossible to give a 100% accurate diagnosis without a full physical examination by a specialized physical therapist or other healthcare provider. Always seek out a qualified healthcare provider for any questions you may have regarding your medical condition.

References

Butler, D. S., & Moseley, L. S. (2003). *Explain Pain*. Adelaide, Noigroup Publications.

Butler. D. S., & Moseley. L. S. (2015). *The Explain Pain Handbook Protectometer*. Adelaide, Noigroup Publications.

Louw, A, Puentedura E (2013). *Therapeutic Neuroscience Education*. Minneapolis, OPTP

Check out **www.noigroup.com** for more great resources to help you better understand why you're feeling what you're feeling.